I0483766

## For more information...

The following free booklets may be helpful if you or your loved one has completed cancer treatment:

*Facing Forward: Life After Cancer Treatment*

*Facing Forward: When Someone You Love Has Completed Cancer Treatment*

These booklets are available from the National Cancer Institute (NCI). To learn more about cancer or to request any of these booklets, visit NCI's Web site, **www.cancer.gov**. You can also call NCI's Cancer Information Service toll-free at 1-800-4-CANCER (1-800-422-6237) to speak with an information specialist.

## Acknowledgments

The National Cancer Institute thanks the many cancer survivors, advocates, and health care professionals who assisted with the development and review of this publication. We would especially like to thank those who gave us their stories to use for this booklet.

# Facing Forward

## Making a Difference in Cancer

Tell me

and I'll forget.

Show me

and I may not remember.

Involve me

and I will understand.

*Chinese proverb*

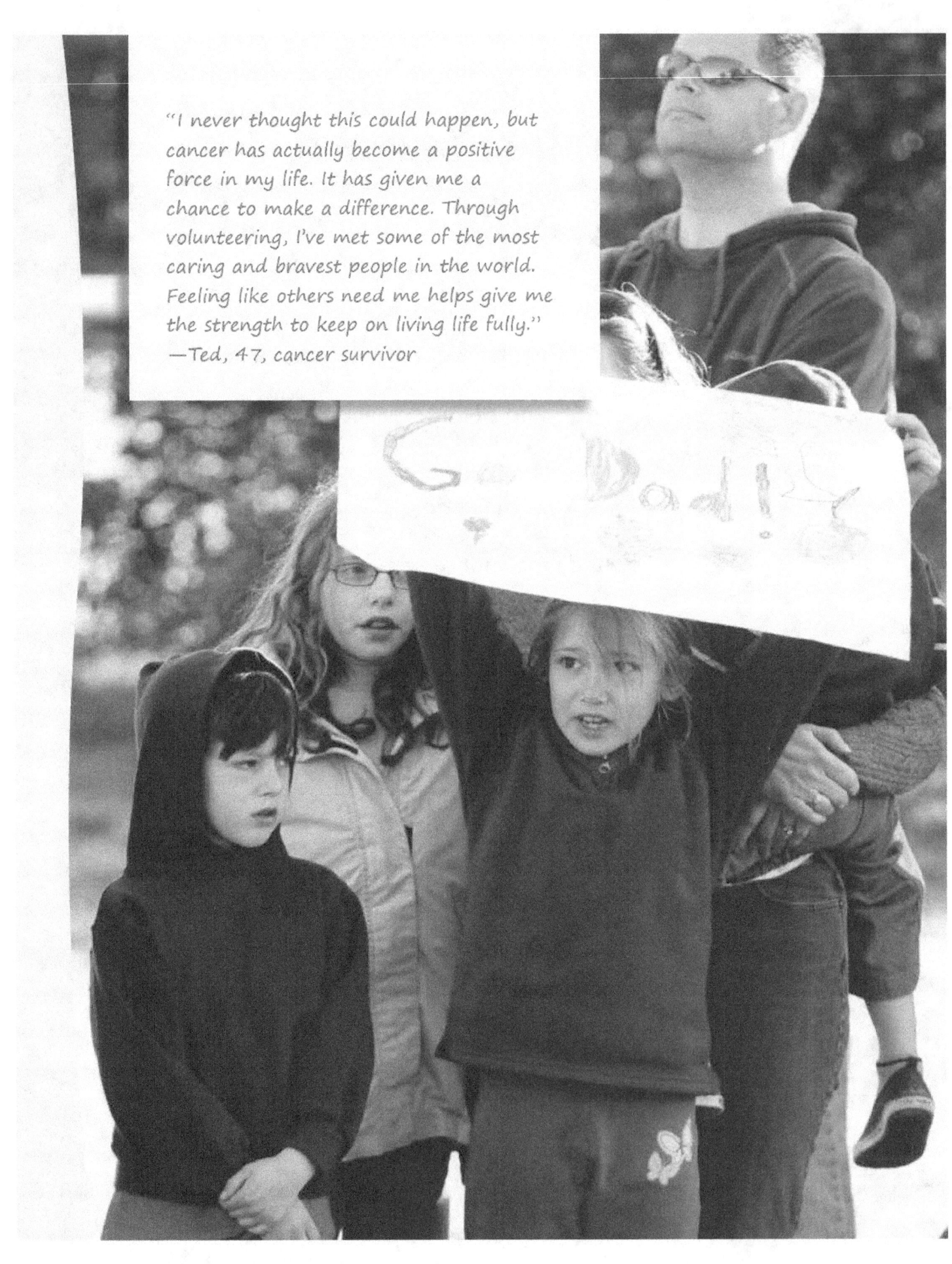

"I never thought this could happen, but cancer has actually become a positive force in my life. It has given me a chance to make a difference. Through volunteering, I've met some of the most caring and bravest people in the world. Feeling like others need me helps give me the strength to keep on living life fully."
—Ted, 47, cancer survivor

# About this booklet

While some people prefer to put their experiences with cancer behind them, many choose to draw on them to get involved with cancer-related activities. They may feel that there are certain areas or issues where there's more work to be done. Or perhaps someone helped and inspired them during treatment, and they feel it's their turn to give to others.

People often feel that they can make a difference in cancer by taking part. They may want to learn how to help their neighbors, join an educational group, run in a race, or be a part of a group that makes decisions about cancer research or programs.

Whether you have cancer or know someone who does, this book has many ideas about ways you can give to others. It's written for anyone who has ever been diagnosed with cancer or affected by it in some way. There are many options for people to choose from: giving support, helping with outreach and education, fundraising, and raising awareness about research or public health issues.

This book may help you:

- **Decide if you want to get involved and volunteer to help others.** Some people are ready right now, while others may choose to devote their energy later. You will need to decide if you're willing to commit your energy and if the time is right for you to start something new.

- **Hear what others have done to take part.** The book has many quotes from people who have taken part in cancer-related activities. We hope they will interest and inspire you.

- **Choose activities that interest you.** This book can help you find things you might like to do. It also has ideas about ways you can put your interests, talents, and skills to good use.

Read this book when the time is right for you. You might want to read only the chapters that interest you now, and then read more later. Or, you may just want to share it with a friend or family member.

## Terms used in this booklet

**Cancer survivor.** A person is considered a cancer survivor from the time of diagnosis onward. Survivors can also be family members or caregivers of people treated for cancer. Not everyone likes the term survivor, but we use it to help people think about their lives as more than just a cancer diagnosis.

**Cancer-related activity.** This refers to any activity that helps others in their cancer experience. This may be a one-time event, like talking on the phone to someone who has cancer. Or it could be done on a regular basis, such as volunteering at a cancer center. It can also be a more long-term activity, like planning a cancer awareness program where you live.

**Advocate.** This is someone who supports, speaks in favor of, or offers suggestions on specific causes. There are many ways to be an advocate, such as being a peer support person, volunteering in a hospital, fundraising, or doing things at a national level.

"My cancer treatment was years ago. At first, I wanted nothing to do with the disease. I wouldn't even read a magazine that had an article about cancer. Now, I'm ready, and I want to help others with my experience."
—Frieda, 72, cancer survivor

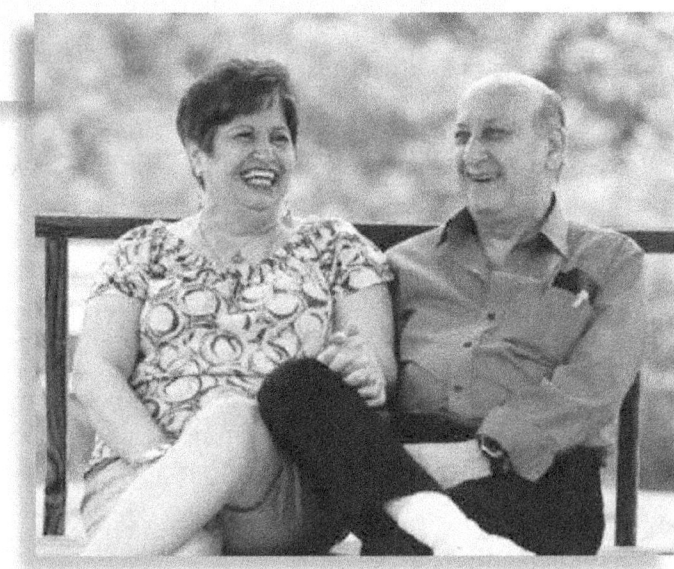

# Table of Contents

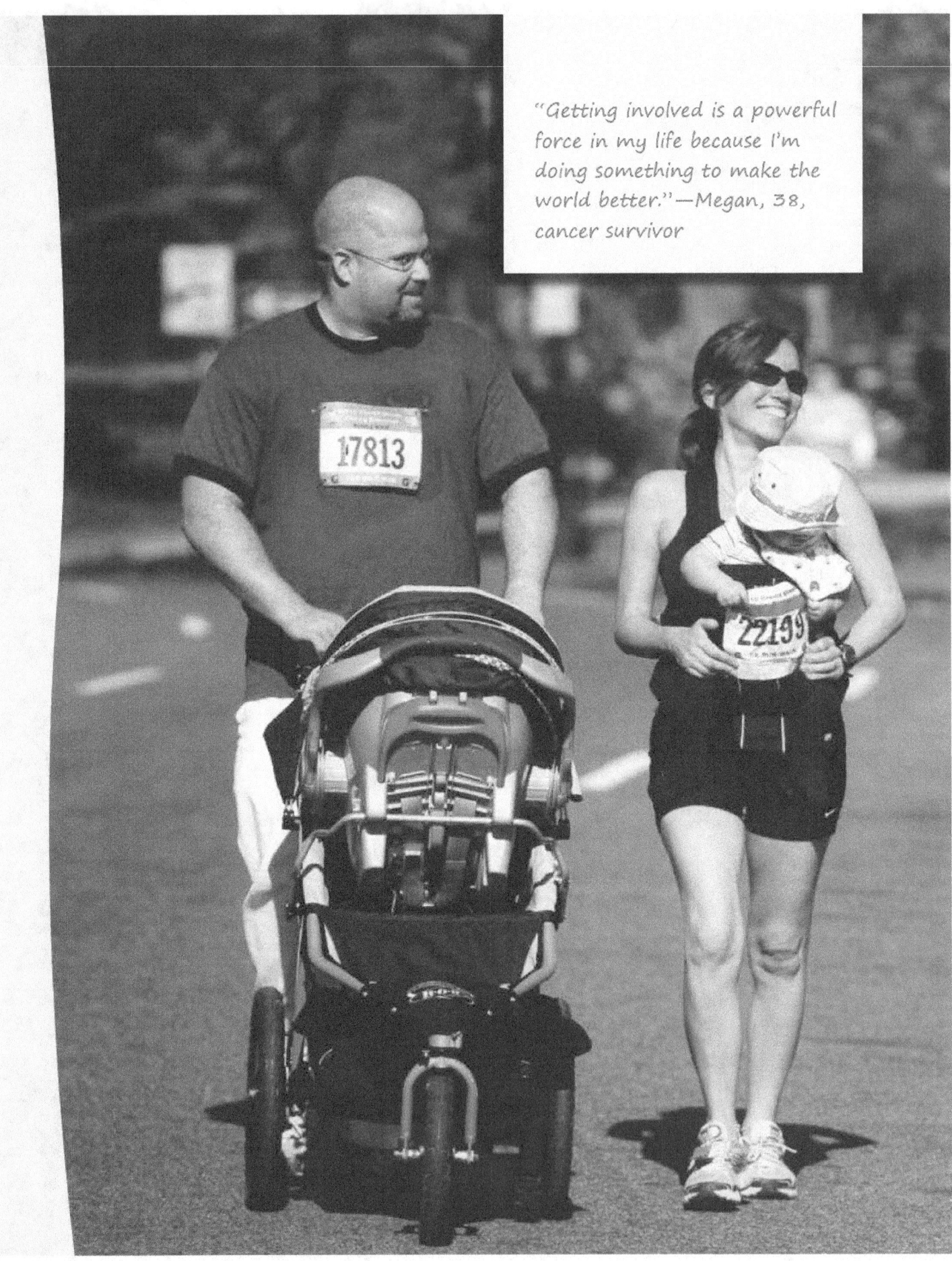

"Getting involved is a powerful force in my life because I'm doing something to make the world better." —Megan, 38, cancer survivor

## Making a difference:
# How you may benefit

Cancer survivors, their loved ones, and others who have lost someone to cancer know what the cancer journey is like. Taking part in cancer-related activities can be a two-way street. Many people find a sense of fulfillment when they help others.

## Common benefits people share:

■ **Accepting cancer as part of life.** For many, getting involved gives new meaning to life.

■ **Being less afraid of cancer.** People often find that the more they know about cancer, the less they fear it.

■ **Learning about cancer.** Some have found that by keeping up with the latest trends and research, they can help others.

■ **Feeling that your cancer experience can serve a purpose and help others.** Research has shown that cancer survivors often find new meaning in their lives when they volunteer. This can be an important part of the healing process.

■ **Having more control in life.** People often feel better when they work with others toward a common goal.

■ **Meeting others who share the same kind of experiences.** People often have a bond with others who have dealt with cancer.

*"Now that I'm a cancer survivor, my life will go on, but it has changed. I want to make my cancer experience mean something."*

*"I can't say I'm glad I got cancer, but I do feel like it gave me a new way of looking at life and a desire to help others like I was helped."*

*"I don't feel like a victim anymore. I've learned to speak up for myself."*

*"It's good to talk to people about what having cancer means to them, as well as help them through it. Only other survivors can really know what it's like."*

1

*Making a difference:*

# Things to think about before you start

People with cancer, as well as those who love and care about them, may want to participate in cancer-related activities. But it's important to ask, **"Is this the right time to get involved?"**

The following questions are for you to think about before taking part in cancer activities. There are no wrong answers, and they may differ for each person. Try to think about what's best for you at this time in your life.

## Am I ready to get involved?

When affected by cancer, volunteering in cancer activities can be a natural reaction for some and a bigger decision for others. It's important to be thoughtful about your reasons for wanting to take part.

**For example, you may not be ready yet if you:**

- Are focused more on your own needs than the needs of others
- Want to talk a lot about your problems with other people
- Feel lonely and want to be with others who understand what you're going through
- Wonder if taking part will be a constant reminder of your cancer

People need time to deal with their feelings and make sense of their cancer experience. If you need to, talk with a counselor, spiritual advisor, psychologist, or your oncology social worker about your feelings and concerns. Joining a support group may help as well. You can always get involved later, when you're truly ready to help others.

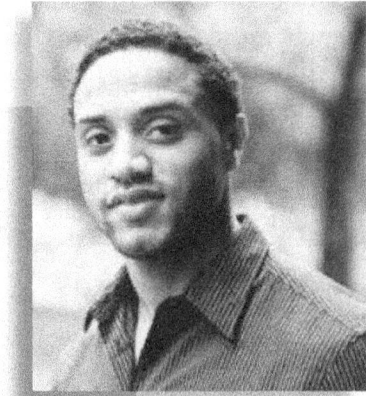

*"Before I started volunteering, I needed to make sure I was ready to help someone else. I knew I couldn't help others if I was still trying to heal myself."*
*—Jason, 32, cancer survivor*

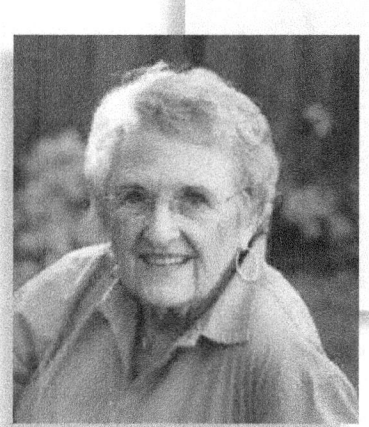

*"I feel every day is special. So once I was well enough, I wanted to start helping others feel this way, too!"*
*—Dotty, 74, cancer survivor*

## How is your health?

Think about your own health issues before you decide to give back. Decide if you have enough energy or time to start a new project. Some people want to wait until their health is better. Others choose something that's easy for them to do now. If you're in treatment or have recently finished, talk to your oncologist before trying something new. If you have advanced cancer, decide if you have the health and strength to get involved right now.

## What are your feelings?

People often think about their own experience when they take part in a cancer-related activity. This is good for some, because it helps them deal with their own feelings. Others find it upsetting. They realize the issues are "too close to home" for them. Or they realize that learning about others' struggles with cancer is hard to bear.

Take some time to think about your feelings. If you tend to feel very worried, angry, or depressed right now, you might want to talk with a counselor or social worker. Later, when you feel better, you can think about ways to help others.

## What are you comfortable talking about?

It's your choice to share what you want to with others about your own experience with cancer. You can still get involved in cancer-related programs even if you don't want to talk about yourself. If this is how you feel, find activities that don't require you to share your personal feelings or thoughts. There are plenty of ideas in this book that may help you.

## What can you give?

Many people feel they don't have a lot of time to volunteer, but there are still ways they can help others. For example, you can donate money, books, or clothing that other people need for their cancer care. Some people even grow their hair out to donate for wigs.

## Where do you live?

If you live in a rural area, or somewhere with no cancer programs nearby, you might have to look for other ways to get involved. You can, for example, start a new project in your community. Or you could plan small gatherings to raise awareness or money. You could also choose to take part in an activity by phone, mail, or over the Internet.

## What are your skills and interests?

What do you like to do with your time? Everyone has an interest or skill that can help others. This includes talents, cultural or spiritual activities, and even your hobbies. Consider what you like, don't like, and subjects you want to learn more about.

Here are some examples of talents or skills that many people have used to make a difference in cancer.

- **Listening.** Let people tell their stories and express their concerns. Answer questions without giving your opinion or advice, trying to solve problems, or passing judgment.

- **Support.** Help others by offering to do errands, baby-sit, or drive them to appointments.

- **Enthusiasm.** Be a cheerleader and motivate others if they need support trying to get things done. With organizations, you could help organize events or work on campaigns. Or, you could help with team sports or outdoor activities for cancer fundraising.

- **Creativity.** Come up with new ideas or use your talents, such as knitting, cooking, building, scrapbooking, or repair work.

- **Technology.** Help people or non-profit organizations develop or enhance a Web site, teach people how to use a computer, or help with Internet searches.

- **Learning and teaching.** Teach or train others in your area of expertise. Take classes to learn new information and then teach others what you know.

- **Communication.** You can get your ideas across by writing cancer-related articles or speaking in public. Or you could have an online diary, called a blog. This is where people post their thoughts and comments to share with others on the Internet.

- **Group work.** Work with others and be part of a team. For example, you could work with your job, school, or place of worship to help raise awareness.

- **Office skills.** Use the computer, answer phones, or organize records and files for a cancer organization or office.

- **Organizational skills.** Plan meetings, events, or group activities, like organizing a phone call alert list or "tree," planning a fundraiser, or starting a local support group.

- **Leadership skills.** Take charge of a program or project. Get people to work together on an activity.

Even if you're not sure about your skills or talents, the next section may give you ideas for what kinds of cancer-related activities will interest and inspire you.

"Whenever somebody says to me, 'I could never get up in front of thousands of people and speak like you do,' I always say, 'You don't have to.'" — Erica, 26, cancer survivor

## Finding ways to make a difference

There are a number of areas where you can find ways to be an advocate in cancer. These include outreach and education, giving support, fundraising, research, or policy issues. Each area may have things you like to do, and that match your interests.

As you read the lists below, think about which items describe you, or note the ones that catch your interest the most. Look at the things that you have experience, skills, or knowledge in doing.

### Helping others

- ■ I like to meet new people.

- ■ I'm good at listening to others.

- ■ I like to share cancer information with others.

- ■ I want to help people who are struggling with cancer.

- ■ People helped me/us during treatment, and now I want to do the same for others.

### Learning and teaching

- ■ I would like to teach people more about cancer.

- ■ I like to talk with people—even people I don't know.

- ■ I like to speak in front of groups of people.

- ■ I enjoy talking about issues that are important to me, like cancer screening or giving support to people with cancer.

### Working on cancer-related events

- ■ I like working with people and being part of events.

- ■ I would like to help with a local event—near where I live or work.

- ■ I want to get involved but only have time to help once in a while.

- ■ I'm comfortable asking people to donate to cancer-related causes.

- I'm interested in giving money, computers, or other items to a cancer-related cause.

- I like having small parties or gatherings.

## Working in policy

- I want to help change the health care system for others with cancer.

- I want to see changes in laws and policies related to cancer.

- I like the idea of talking to elected officials about cancer issues.

- I like to share my ideas with others through phone calls, letters, or e-mails.

- I want to be part of a network that alerts people to important cancer issues.

## Working in research

- I find science very interesting.

- I may be interested in taking part in a research study or clinical trial.

- I want to let others know about research studies and clinical trials.

- I like the idea of talking with scientists about my opinions on cancer, and my experiences with it.

## Working in government programs

- I want to work on programs that help people with cancer.

- I would like to help more people get screened for cancer.

- I think I would be comfortable talking about cancer with scientists and public health officials.

- I would like to know how new medicines and treatments are developed and approved.

# Making a difference:
## Everyday ways

There are many ways you can help others. This chapter looks at how you can make a difference in everyday ways, like helping someone with daily tasks, learning and teaching, sharing your experiences, or helping others through the health care system.

## Helping with daily activities

You can make a big difference in small ways. This includes day-to-day things such as chores and errands. For example, you can:

- Help people with their grocery shopping or household chores.

- Offer to baby-sit their children or take care of their pets. You could also offer to take the kids out for awhile.

- Drive people to their doctors' appointments. This can be a big help, especially when people have to travel a long distance.

- Arrange meals, do errands, or mow the lawn for someone who is sick. "We decided to help organize meals after our neighbor got five pans of lasagna in one day," said a friend of someone with colon cancer.

- Do things for others that you would have liked people to have done for you.

"Giving back has helped my recovery. It gave me something to do and took my mind off what I was going through. I was able to get involved and get moving. When I'm helping others, I don't have time to think about myself or have any self-pity."
—Vince, 40, cancer survivor

■ Help them with repair work or other home projects if you're handy with tools.

■ Read books aloud to others or make a music CD for them.

■ If you enjoy crafts such as knitting or quilting, you can donate scarves and blankets for patients going through chemotherapy or radiation.

## Sharing your experiences

If you're reading this book, you probably know that your experience can help others who are struggling. Here are some ways you can help:

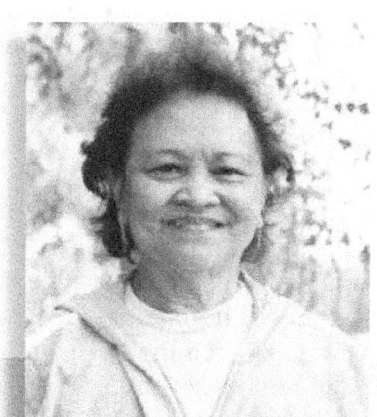

■ Offer to be a "buddy" to someone who is dealing with cancer. You can do this in person, by telephone, or even over the Internet. Many cancer organizations have support programs that meet online.

■ Ask how you can be helpful to the family and friends of someone who has cancer. Let them know that you care and are ready to listen, help, and share ideas.

■ Become a trained "peer counselor." This is someone who is trained to help others with the same type of experience or diagnosis. Keep in mind that some cancer organizations suggest, or even require, that people be out of treatment for at least a year before they begin.

*"It took me 3 years to set up a local survivors' group in my area. My support group started with two people in my home and grew to ten. I think it's important to help people so that they can heal and recover." —Irma, 59, cancer survivor*

■ Get involved with, or start, a cancer support group in your area.

■ Let people know where they can learn more about cancer (see next page). Share helpful resources from the National Cancer Institute or other cancer organizations with them.

# Learning more about cancer

When you learn about cancer, you not only help yourself, but you can also help others by sharing what you know. For example, you can learn about your rights as a person with cancer and share this with others. Or you can help people in their search for information. Here are some ways to get started:

## By phone

Many national cancer organizations have toll-free phone numbers. They can answer your questions or send you materials with more information. Some cancer organizations conduct educational programs over the telephone.

## In print

There is a lot of written information about cancer in magazines, newspapers, booklets, and books. Some of these print materials are written for the general public, while others are for health professionals and scientists. Visit your local library or hospital resource center, or ask your doctor or nurse about up-to-date materials that are written at the right level for you. Many print materials can be accessed online now as well.

## Going to meetings, workshops, or classes

Many people help themselves as well as others by going to meetings, workshops, and classes. They can learn about clinical trials, ways to relax, or how to cope with other problems that come up after treatment is over. Ask your local hospital or cancer center about cancer-related programs they offer the general public. Often, you can attend these programs for free or at a low cost.

"There's a new study published every day. I want to keep up with the information my wife needs." —Ray, husband of a 66-year-old breast cancer survivor

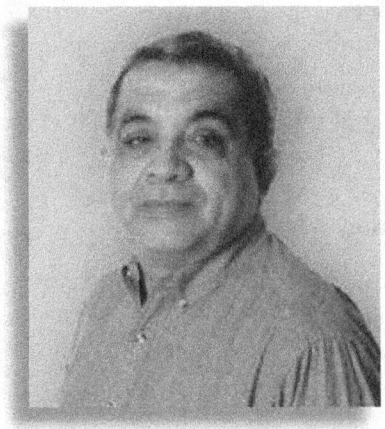

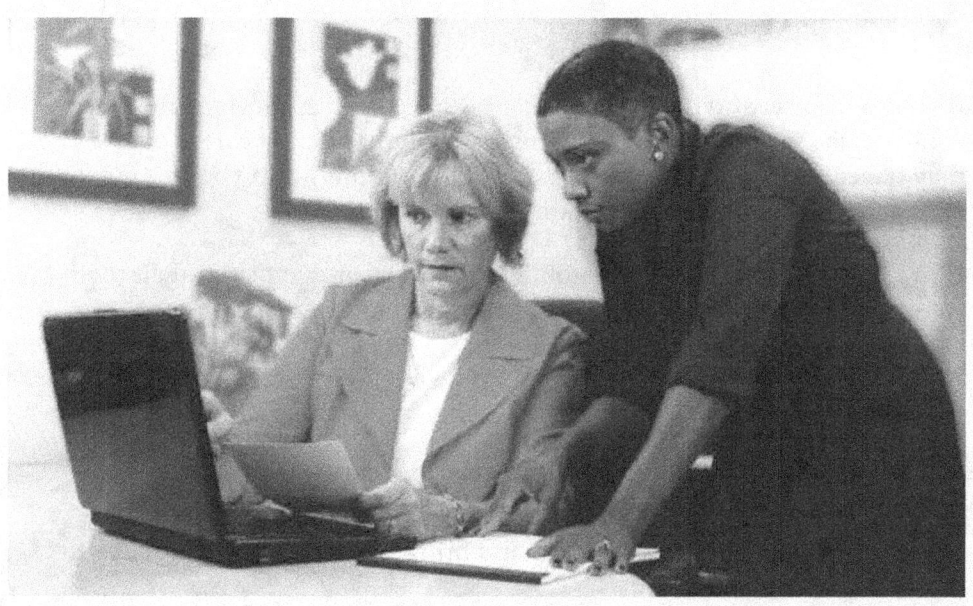

## Over the Internet

Many people search for cancer information on the Internet. Most organizations have Web sites you can go to for the latest information about cancer. You may also want to make use of social media. This involves social contact through Web sites such as Facebook, Twitter, and others.

You could subscribe to an organization's e-mail list and get messages when the site is updated. Some have **RSS Feeds** that you can sign up for, which allows you to receive breaking news alerts in the cancer area.

Some Web sites offer listservs or chat rooms where people can meet and talk online. These are ways that people interested in cancer can exchange messages about their experiences, concerns, and resources.

If you don't have access to the Internet at home, you may be able to use computers at your local library. Or ask your doctor, librarian, or a family member or friend to help you find information. You can also call NCI's Cancer Information Service at 1-800-4-CANCER and ask them to mail you information from NCI's Web site.

Remember: The Internet can be a valuable source of information about cancer. But sometimes the information can be false, unreliable, or misleading. Don't believe everything you see on the Internet. Also, check the privacy statements and settings of the social media sites before signing up. Talk with your doctor about the medical advice you find and make sure the information makes sense for you. To learn more, see the NCI fact sheet *Evaluating Health Information on the Internet* at **http://www.cancer.gov/cancertopics/factsheet/Information/internet**.

## Helping with health care providers

If you're a cancer survivor or are close to someone with cancer, you know what it's like to talk with doctors, nurses, and other health care providers. You may have learned how to speak up and ask questions—and you can use your experience to help others. For example, you can:

■ Let people know that they should talk with their doctor about all their concerns—even the ones they may not think are important.

■ Direct them to resources that help people learn ways to talk with their health care team.

■ Help patients and their families get ready for medical appointments. You can suggest that they:

- Write a list of their questions and bring it with them when they see the doctor.

- Have pen and paper to take notes about what the doctor says.

- Bring a friend or family member with them to their appointments to take notes or help listen.

- Provide a folder or file for any relevant tests. Encourage them to keep it up to date and bring it to every visit.

### Going to the doctor

If you offer to go to a doctor's appointment with someone, make sure you agree on what he or she would like you to do. Ask ahead of time if you should:

■ Stay in the waiting area or go into the exam room with the patient.

■ Ask questions or help explain any words or terms that are hard to understand.

■ Bring paper and pen or a tape recorder to take notes.

■ Offer to sit with the patient or their caregiver during treatment to keep them company.

## Ways others have helped where they live

■ A breast cancer survivor saw a need for other patients to know they're not alone. With funding from her local hospital and donations from area merchants, she made kits to give to women going through cancer treatment. Each kit contains comforting items and information about services in the area.

■ Members of a cancer support group were trained to help at a local hospice. They gave comfort to patients and showed kindness to their friends and family members.

■ Older, trusted members of one community reached out to their neighbors about cancer screening. Known as "lay health advisors," they encouraged other older adults to get screened for cancer.

■ A hospital organized a "Patient Navigator Program" in which survivors helped people who had cancer but did not have health insurance. They worked together throughout the person's cancer treatment.

■ To cope with his grief over his wife's death from lung cancer, one man began sewing quilts in his spare time. To reach people beyond his small town, he decided to auction them over the Internet. As he continues to sew and sell his quilts, he's also found comfort by donating all the proceeds to lung cancer research.

■ Some groups have found ways to help others who share their faith, background, or culture. A group of African-American women with cancer organized a support group to deal with their unique needs. And a local church started a program to spread the message about the importance of early breast cancer detection.

■ One man used his love of taking pictures and his cancer experience to inspire others. He designed a calendar with peaceful nature photos and quotes of hope to give out to cancer patients in his state.

## How to begin helping in everyday ways

Once you decide that you want to volunteer your time, find out who needs your help and what you can do to get started. Here are some ideas about ways to begin:

■ **Let people know that you want to help others.** Tell your family, friends, coworkers, and even your health care team that you want to get involved in cancer-related activities. Talk with them about things you like to do and ways you want to help. Ask for their ideas and suggestions.

■ **Look at Web resources for setting up communication sites.** If you're good with computers, offer to set up a blog or Web page where friends and family can be updated on the patient's progress.

■ **Find out about volunteer programs where you live.** Check with your local hospital or cancer center, clubs, libraries, senior centers, and places of worship to see if they have programs to help people with cancer. If any of these groups have volunteer programs, ask how you can get involved. If there isn't a program nearby, perhaps you could start one.

■ **Get involved with a cancer organization.** Contact a cancer-related group that interests you. Talk with the person in charge of volunteers about your interests and experiences.

■ **Join a Patient and Family Advisory Board.** Hospitals and cancer centers often want survivors and their families to help them develop new programs. When you are on a Patient and Family Advisory Board, you may be asked to give advice on policies and programs and let the organization know how it can improve care for all patients.

## Making a difference:
# Cancer-related organizations

Cancer-related organizations include many different kinds of groups that help people with cancer. Many of them need the help of volunteers. Some programs serve only their local communities, while others help people in certain regions of the country. National organizations serve people all across the United States.

### Cancer-related organizations can focus on different areas:

- All types of cancer
- Just one type of cancer
- One topic, such as prevention, treatment, support, or survivorship
- The needs of people from a specific racial or ethnic group, religion, or culture
- The needs of family members or other people who take care of those with cancer

### They also can focus on different types of advocacy areas:

- Service and support
- Fundraising
- Research
- Policy/political

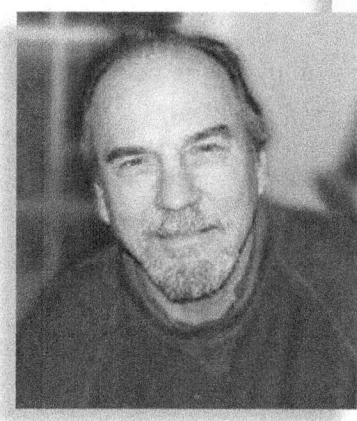

"After my sister died of lung cancer, I started pitching in for a local organization that was raising money for cancer research. I channeled all my feelings into volunteering. I have made some great friends and helped raise money, too."—Tom, 54, lost a sister to cancer

Think about your interests, and decide if you want to volunteer with a cancer-related organization that helps people with the issues mentioned above. You can also decide if you want to help others who live in your own area, or those who live across the United States. See below for the many options for you to choose.

## Working with service and support organizations

Service and support organizations raise awareness about cancer and also ensure that people don't have to face it alone. They offer help to the public, survivors, caregivers, and people who lost someone to cancer. These groups provide services such as:

- **Education.** Teaching people about screening tests, ways to reduce cancer risks, and healthy living tips, are some of the ways organizations educate about cancer. They often give workshops and presentations at workplaces, schools, places of worship, health fairs, and even over the phone or Internet.

- **Online help.** Many organizations have volunteers who are trained to answer questions on the Internet. Some may answer your questions within a certain time period. Others are able to have real-time text chats with you online.

- **Awareness.** Many organizations hold events like runs or walks, fundraisers, health fairs and screenings, and information booths. They can often use your help to make sure things run smoothly.

- **Telephone hotlines.** In these programs, volunteers are trained to be hotline counselors, people who give easy-to-understand information over the phone. They're also trained to be good listeners and support other people as they talk about their feelings and concerns. Some hotlines let volunteers conduct calls from their homes.

- **Cancer support programs.** These programs give emotional support to people with cancer and their families. They also help by giving people items they need, such as wigs, scarves, books, and DVDs.

- **Other types of support.** Some organizations help with medical services, including referrals for second opinions or specialists. They also include legal and financial services, as well as the practical help people need, like rides to medical appointments. Or you could be a greeter or host in hospitals, or at the help desk.

## Working with fundraising organizations

All cancer organizations have to raise money to provide the services people need and want. Many groups also raise funds for cancer research.

Fundraising is often done through activities such as sporting events or shows. These events not only bring in money, but also raise awareness about cancer and give hope to the people who participate.

### Types of fundraising events

There are many kinds of fundraising events. They may raise money for cancer screening, outreach, education, or research. You could even hold an event on a smaller scale in your community, or host one in your home.

Here are some examples:

- Walks, runs, and races. Many of these events take place on weekends; some take two or three days to complete.

- Activities like golf, bowling, cycling, and dancing

- Luncheons, dinners, auctions, and fashion shows

- Plays and concerts

## How to help with fundraising events

- Take part in an event, and encourage others to do the same.

- Organize an event in your community.

- Buy a ticket or make a donation to an event.

- Donate food or items for raffles or auctions.

- Sponsor someone to take part in a race or game.

- Help think of new ways to raise money and find volunteers to work on events.

- Help with writing press releases or promotional items.

## What you should know

■ Every organization that raises money needs to publish its budget and annual report. The organization has to state where the funds go and how much is given to cancer-related activities.

■ Find out ahead of time how the organization plans to use the money you raise. You might want to ask:

- How will the money be spent? Will it focus on local or national programs?

- Who decides how the money will be spent?

- What percent of the money goes to helping people with cancer?

- Does the event support all types of cancer or just one type?

For more information, see the NCI fact sheet, *Cancer Fund-Raising Organizations*, at **www.cancer.gov/cancertopics/factsheet**. Or you may call the NCI Cancer Information service at 1-800-4-CANCER and ask for a copy.

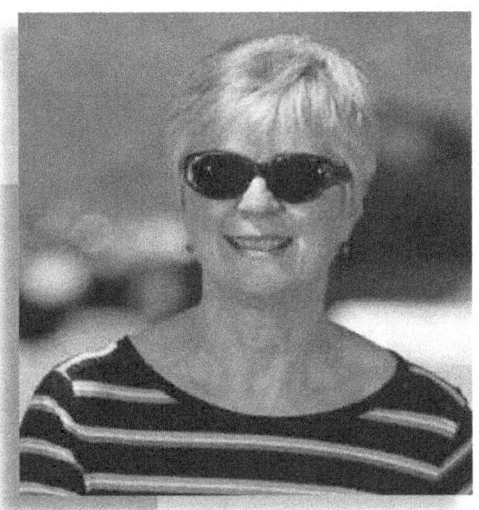

"Each year, my friends and I form a team for our local cancer awareness walk. We all have loved ones who have had the disease, so it's a way of giving back."
—Patti, 58, lost her father to cancer

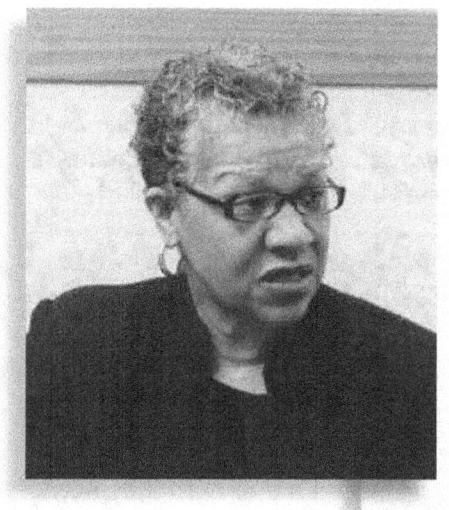

"We've educated elected officials about our struggles with cancer, and I've gotten my support group to gather lots of signatures on our latest petition drive. It makes me feel that I'm making a difference for others who will face this disease." —Connie, 62, cancer advocate

## Working to influence policy

Some people like to get involved with influencing government policy. There are cancer organizations that do this by supporting or speaking in favor of certain causes. For example:

■ Helping people with cancer get the care they need, even if they don't have health insurance or can't pay for it.

■ Protecting people from being treated unfairly because they have cancer or other health-related problems.

■ Raising awareness about cancer, and talking to people about the need for more services, education, and research.

## How to get started in political issues

- **Become an active, involved citizen and consumer.** For example, you can join a city, state, or regional effort to get more people involved in cancer policy issues. You can also speak about these issues at meetings, health fairs, and other public events.

- **Get to know your elected officials** and talk with them about your cancer concerns.

- **Sign a petition on cancer issues.** Advocacy groups often use petitions as a way to bring attention to cancer issues.

- **Join a politically focused committee** and see what kind of help they need. They may ask you to make phone calls, write letters, or organize an event. If there isn't a group near you, see if you can help by making phone calls or sending emails for them.

- **Sign up to receive cancer "alert" announcements.** Many advocacy groups mail, fax, or e-mail alerts about important cancer issues. Use these to keep up to date, and ask your friends and neighbors if they want to get this information as well.

## Finding cancer-related organizations

- Find cancer-related organizations by going to the Resources list on page 27. Many of these groups have local chapters. You can also find local groups by calling your local hospital, your oncology clinic, searching the Internet, or asking a friend, neighbor, or someone at your doctor's office.

- Contact organizations that interest you and ask for information about their programs. Start by going to one of their events or talking with someone who organizes volunteers. See if there is a good fit between your interests and what they do.

- Contact the health department or a hospital in your area. They should have suggestions of what organizations would be helpful to you.

*Making a difference:*

# Cancer research

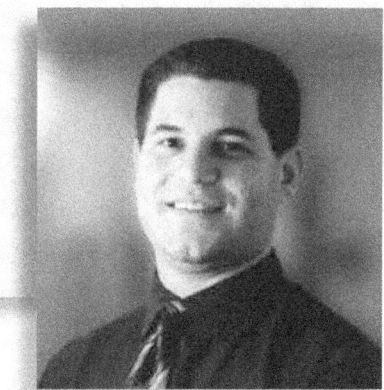

"After my brother finished treatment for colon cancer, I wanted to take part in something that might help others in some way. The cancer center's patient education office told me about a colon cancer prevention study that was taking place. The trial compares different diets that might reduce the risk for getting the disease. It's been really easy to take part, and I feel like I'm making a difference, too!" —Chris, 47, brother of cancer survivor

## Taking part in cancer research

Research is the key to improving prevention, detection, and treatment for cancer. The treatments and interventions that will be used in the future are being developed based on the people who take part in research studies today. The more people join, the sooner we may find more options for cancer control.

Cancer research takes place at hospitals, universities, government facilities, private companies, and in the community. There are different ways you can get involved, such as spreading the word about the benefits of research, taking part in it, encouraging others to do so, and helping to influence how research is done.

### Joining a research study

Clinical trials are research studies that involve people. These studies help doctors find ways to improve cancer care. Each trial tries to answer scientific questions and find better ways to prevent, diagnose, or treat cancer.

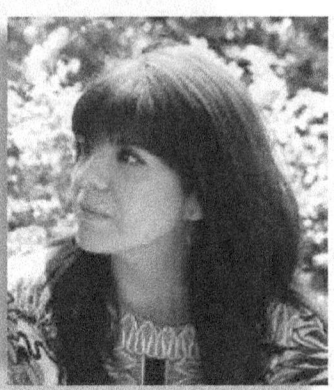

"My 13-year old son died of cancer. So I have a unique viewpoint to share. And as an advocate, I help doctors and scientists understand what parents of children with cancer go through."—Juana, 40, lost her son to cancer

**You don't have to have cancer to take part in a trial.** Cancer treatment trials test whether a new drug or procedure is effective. But if you're a cancer survivor, or a friend or family member of someone affected by cancer, there are many options to try. For example, there are:

■ Clinical trials that focus on cancer prevention, cancer screening, or health behavior.

■ Research studies that ask survivors and their families to fill out surveys or take part in interviews. These studies may focus on understanding more about:

- The things people do or are exposed to that may affect their health

- How cancer affected their lives

- The medical costs of cancer and its treatment

Taking part in a research study—once you learn all you should about it—may be an important way to give to others and, perhaps, yourself as well. You can find more information below.

## To learn more about clinical trials:

To find clinical trials that are right for you, contact the National Cancer Institute (NCI) at 1-800-4-CANCER, or go to: **http://www.cancer.gov/clinicaltrials.**

For example, you can:

■ Learn more about how clinical trials have helped find better treatments for people with cancer.

■ Find out how you can teach others about participating in these studies.

■ Find out where clinical trials are taking place in your area.

■ Talk to your doctor about clinical trials in your area. Some of these studies may also be listed in your local newspaper.

## Having a voice in cancer research funding

Before designing a study, scientists and health care experts need to decide what topics to research, how the research will be done, and how it will be funded. And it's not just doctors and scientists in lab coats who think about these issues.

People who have had cancer and others who are concerned about the disease are starting to have a voice in how research is funded. Often called *consumer* or *patient advocates*, they bring a vital point of view to the research process. They can explain what is really important to people who have cancer. Patient advocates also help scientists know what it's like for patients to take part in cancer research.

When deciding what projects to fund, whether sponsored by a private organization, a state government, or the federal government, cancer research programs must review applications to look for the ones that show the most promise. For example:

- Many foundations raise money for cancer research, education, and outreach programs and then award funds to projects they feel are worthy.

- Many states, as well as the federal government, award funds to scientists for cancer research.

Some of these programs invite people to join committees that help decide which research gets funded. These advocates can bring a community perspective to such important decisions. By serving on these committees, reviewers help gather support for:

- New research studies that will benefit patients sooner and more effectively

- Improved medical care

- Improved quality of life for patients, survivors, and their families

There are a number of different programs that seek advocate input into what research gets funded. See the Resources list on page 27 for more information.

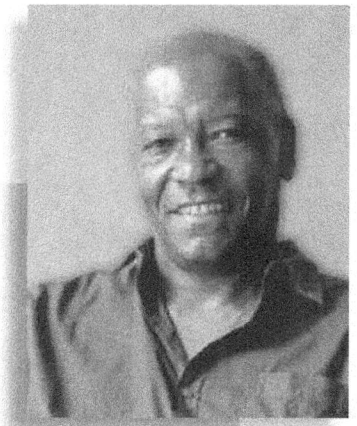

*"I like speaking in front of people and being able to stand up for others. So becoming a reviewer felt natural to me." —Howard, 68, cancer survivor*

## Joining an institutional review board

Another way you can get involved in research is by joining an institutional review board (IRB) at your local hospital, cancer center, or university. An IRB is made up of doctors, nurses, and people from the community. Its job is to review research studies and make sure they are run in a manner that is safe and fair. IRB members also look at informed consent documents and ensure that they are easy to understand. They also verify that they contain the information people should know about the study.

## To learn more about having a voice in cancer research:

- Contact the research office at your local hospital, university, or cancer center. Ask to speak with the researchers to learn more about their work.

- Learn about research in your community by visiting the NCI Funded Research Portfolio Web site at: **http://fundedresearch.cancer.gov**. You can search this site by state, institution, or name of researcher.

- Contact your state's health department and ask about the cancer research programs it funds. Find out which studies are looking for members of the public to get involved in some way.

- Contact the cancer organizations listed in the Resources section on page 27 to find out the ways they involve people affected by cancer.

- To find local cancer programs, look on the Internet or in your telephone book under "Departments of Health" or "Health Departments."

- Learn about the private foundations in your area that fund cancer research, and show them the value of a patient perspective. Ask them if they accept advocate input.

*Making a difference:*

# Government programs

## Working with government programs

Survivors and their families can make a difference in the types of programs the government offers to people with cancer (or people at risk for developing cancer). They can bring an important community perspective to government.

### There are three levels of government cancer programs:

- **Local.** Many county and city health departments have cancer education, awareness, and screening programs. To ensure that programs work well, these departments often ask survivors and their family members to get involved. For example, a local health department might ask for advice about what types of projects should go forward.

- **State.** States also offer programs to improve cancer care and reduce cancer deaths. These programs may focus on cancer education, prevention, early detection, or treatment. For example, a state may run a program educating older men about prostate cancer.

- **National.** Just as local governments need the advice of consumers, the federal government has several programs that benefit from the advice of cancer survivors and their families. For example, cancer advocates may provide input when cancer funding efforts are prioritized, by participating on committees or reviewing research proposals.

## How to get started in government programs

Decide if you want to get involved at the local, state, or national level. You may want to start out in your home county. **Be aware that it may take time to get involved at the state or national level.** You often have to put in both hard work and time to make contacts and connections. However, for those who are willing, it can be very rewarding.

If you think you may be interested in government cancer programs, a good way to start is by speaking with the person in charge of cancer-related programs at your local health department or hospital. Ask for information about the programs they offer and find out how you can help. To find out about:

- **National programs.** Look at the Resources section on page 27. If an organization interests you, call, write a letter, or look at their Web site for more information or to request an application. Keep in mind that at this level, they may only work with advocates who have specific experience or a history in advocacy.

- **State cancer programs.** Speak to someone who works on cancer in your state health department. Ask for information about their programs and find out how you can help. Or contact the Centers for Disease Control and Prevention (CDC) at 1-800-232-4636 or **http://www.cdc.gov/cancer/dcpc/ about/programs.htm**.

- **Local cancer programs.** Look in your telephone book or go to your city or county's local Web site. Look for "Departments of Health" or "Health Departments" to get started. You could also call your local hospital or cancer organization.

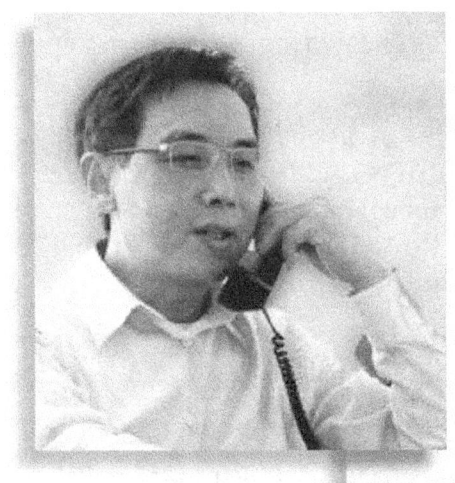

"After my cancer treatment I started going to meetings, and got information that I passed along to others. Later on, I was asked to be on a government committee about funding for cancer research. Since then, I've been on lots of government committees. When I'm working with these groups, I try to speak up for others facing cancer."—Lee, 47, cancer survivor

# Resources

**For a complete list of resources:**

See the database, *National Organizations That Offer Cancer-Related Services*, at **www.cancer.gov**, using the search terms "national organizations." Or call 1-800-4-CANCER (1-800-422-6237) to ask for it.

The following list includes national organizations that provide information support and other resources to cancer patients, survivors, and those who have helped someone through cancer. Many of these groups have volunteer opportunities in your community, or at the state or national level. There are many other organizations that are disease- or population-specific. See the box to the right for more information.

## Federal organizations

■ **National Cancer Institute (NCI)**
Provides comprehensive, research-based information on cancer prevention, screening, diagnosis, treatment, genetics, and supportive care.
**Web site:**      www.cancer.gov

### NCI's Cancer Information Service (CIS)
CIS answers questions about cancer, clinical trials, and cancer-related services and helps users find information on the NCI Web site. It also provides NCI printed materials.
**Phone:**          1-800-4-CANCER (1-800-422-6237)
**Web site:**      www.cancer.gov/aboutnci/cis
**Chat online:**  www.cancer.gov/livehelp

### Office of Advocacy Relations (OAR)
NCI's Office of Advocacy Relations (OAR) engages the advocacy and NCI communities by communicating with them about cancer research programs and priorities. OAR involves individuals in the research process in a number of areas.
**Phone:**          301-594-3194
**Web site:**      advocacy.cancer.gov

■ **U.S. Department of Defense Congressionally Directed Medical Research Programs (CDMRP)**

CDMRP oversees cancer research programs in which patient/consumer reviewers take part in reviewing research proposals along with scientists.

**Phone:**      301-619-7079

**E-mail:**      cdmrpconsumers@amedd.army.mil

**Web site:**   cdmrp.army.mil

■ **Food and Drug Administration (FDA)**

Several FDA Programs involve patient and consumer representatives in FDA's drug review process. The following Web sites provide information on the programs, how to find out more, and how to apply:

**Patient Representatives:**

www.fda.gov/ForConsumers/ByAudience/ForPatientAdvocates

**Consumer Representatives:**

www.fda.gov/AdvisoryCommittees/AboutAdvisoryCommittees/
CommitteeMembership/ApplyingforMembership/default.htm

## Nonprofit organizations

■ **American Cancer Society (ACS)**

ACS's mission is to end cancer as a major health problem through prevention, saving lives, and relieving suffering. ACS works toward these goals through research, education, advocacy, and service. The organization's National Cancer Information Center answers questions 24 hours a day, 7 days a week.

**Phone:**      1-800-ACS-2345 (1-800-227-2345)

**TTY:**        1-866-228-4327

**Web site:**   www.cancer.org

■ **CancerCare**

CancerCare provides free, professional support services, including counseling, education, financial assistance, and practical help.

**Phone:**      1-800-813-HOPE (1-800-813-4673)

**Web site:**   www.cancercare.org

■ **Cancer Hope Network**

Cancer Hope Network matches patients and families with trained volunteers who have recovered from a similar cancer experience.

**Phone:** 1-877-HOPENET (1-877-467-3638)

**Web site:** www.cancerhopenetwork.org

■ **Cancer Support Community (CSC)**

The CSC is dedicated to providing support, education, and hope to people affected by cancer.

**Phone:** 1-888-793-9355

**Web site:** www.cancersupportcommunity.org

■ **Family Caregiver Alliance (FCA)**

FCA addresses the needs of families and friends who provide long-term care at home.

**Phone:** 1-800-445-8106

**Web site:** www.caregiver.org

■ **Lance Armstrong Foundation (LAF)**

LAF seeks to inspire and empower people living with, through, and beyond cancer to live strong. It provides education, advocacy, and public health and research programs.

**Phone:** 1-512-236-8820 (general number)

1-866-235-7205 (LIVESTRONG SurvivorCare program)

**Web site:** www.livestrong.org

■ **National Coalition for Cancer Survivorship (NCCS)**

NCCS provides information and resources on cancer support, advocacy, and quality-of-life issues to cancer survivors and their loved ones. They offer online advocacy training and materials.

**Phone:** 1-877-NCCS-YES (1-877-622-7937)

**Web site:** www.canceradvocacy.org

■ **National Family Caregivers Association (NFCA)**

NFCA provides information, education, support, public awareness, and advocacy for caregivers.

**Phone:** 1-800-896-3650

**Web site:** www.nfcacares.org

■ **National Hospice and Palliative Care Organization (NHPCO)**

NHPCO provides information on hospice care, local hospice programs, state-specific advance directives, and locating a local health care provider. NHPCO also provides educational materials on palliative and end-of-life issues, as well as links to other organizations and resources.

**Toll-free:**    1-800-658-8898

**Visit:**        www.nhpco.org

### Caring Connections

Caring Connections is a program of the NHPCO to educate consumers and engage the public to improve care at the end of life.

**Toll-free:**  1-800-658-8898

**Visit:**      www.caringinfo.org

■ **Patient Advocate Foundation (PAF)**

PAF provides education, legal counseling, and referrals to cancer patients and survivors. It specializes in matters related to managed care, insurance, financial issues, job discrimination, and debt crisis.

**Phone:**      1-800-532-5274

**Web site:**   www.patientadvocate.org